Diet 66

Ben Harris

Books by Ben Harris

Fiction:

- The adventure of Harry and George in the illusion of time
- The Little girl and the tiger cub
- Wrath of the Empire

Non-fiction:

- You're number 1
- Diet 66

If you're a passionate reader and interested in becoming a beta reader with free access to early releases, then reach out by email. I would love to have you on board.

For more information

Contact: BenjaminHarris@gmx.com

First published in Great Britain in 2020 by Ben Harris

2 3 4 5 6 7 8 9 10 1

First printed and bound in Great Britain in 2020 by Ben Harris

ISBN 9798656990059

The second book by Ben Harris

"Thou should eat to live; not live to eat."

— Socrates

Introduction

Diet 66 – is a step-by-step guide covering a vast range of areas around food and active healthy living. It covers 66 individual topics, giving you guidance to get you to the ultimate body of your dreams. Just following one of these points can give you significant progress. Implementing more than one will be better. The more you do, the more you will get out of it. The guide is meant to be based on your current habits. It is for you to pick and choose which elements best suit you. Ideally, the ones which you find easiest to put in place and maintain. The book is designed so that you can skip to any section. You do not have to read from start to finish. That way, you can go to what you need right now and then move onto the next section when you are ready. Each section is only 1-4 pages with a view to keeping it simple and straightforward to take in and implement. Changes should not be complex or difficult for you to achieve. They should also be minimal to make it easier for you. As human beings' minds go on autopilot. Which means we get stuck in routine easily and find it difficult to change. So small steady steps and just take the sections that you want to put in place. Do not dare do anything that you will find difficult or will be unable to maintain. This book is for you to get results and to win. Any other way or feelings towards the change and you will most likely fail. So, do what you want and not one anyone else tells you to do. Just do it with knowledge and the information to support you. So, you can make a wise decision. "Whatever you do, never give up. As the second you do, you lose." "It's okay to fail, as long as you go back to it, again and again. Change your approach and you will eventually win.

To start, read and implement Step 1, after that pick 3 other steps and get them in place for 4-8 weeks. Keep going until you stop making progress, then add another 2-4 steps, then repeat.

Start with the introduction before chapter 1

1. One change
2. Alcohol
3. Desserts
4. Breakfast
5. Lunch
6. Dinner
7. Supper
8. Snacks
9. Water
10. Coffee, tea, and hot drinks
11. Protein
12. Fats
13. Carbs
14. Vitamins
15. Supplements
16. Dairy
17. Sweets
18. Chocolate
19. Cakes
20. Biscuits
21. Takeaway food
22. Eating out
23. Peer pressure
24. Juice
25. Milk
26. Movement

27. Exercise
28. Stretching
29. Weightlifting
30. Cardio
31. Exercise classes
32. Calories
33. Sports Drinks
34. Veggie + Vegan diets
35. Fruit
36. Vegetables
37. Nuts and seeds
38. Eggs
39. Planning and shopping
40. Food preparation
41. Food labels information
42. Meat
43. Fish
44. Fasting
45. Food swaps
46. Food diaries
47. Feeling of food – before and after
48. Eating on holiday
49. Benefits of healthy eating
50. Keeping a balance
51. Mind and thinking right
52. Body and taking care of yourself
53. Downtime – preventing burn out

54. Goal setting
55. Body stats and measurements
56. Reviewing progress
57. Personal trainers
58. Exercising at home
59. Cereals
60. Frozen food
61. Time
62. Travel
63. Eating for reasons
64. Implementing your plan
65. Barriers
66. Results, winning the game

Summary

Step 1 - One change

This step is all about making just one change in your life. Most importantly, one change in your diet. It can be implemented in life, but the focus here is on diet. The change should be easy, and it should be manageable. It should also be a change that you want to make. Your take on it should be to see the change as the better option of the two. Rather than sticking with it. So, for example, if you love chocolate, then there is no way in hell you are taking it out of your diet. Whereas if you do not mind it and just have it for the sake of it. The better option might be the results you get from removing it from your diet. Now, this section is about making a change, not necessarily removing anything from your life.

So, what I want you to do for this section is to think about or write out the food and drink that you eat on a daily basis. Not food and drink you have on a weekly basis. So, this might be tea, coffee, breakfast cereal, toast, or a banana, for example. I then want you to find out how many calories are in the food and drink you have listed. This can be done with the help of an internet search engine or a calorie counting app. Now it should not be lots of calorie counting. It is just looking at some of your daily food and drink, say no more than 4 or 5 different items.

Some examples:

- Banana, medium - 105 calories (kcal).

- Latte, medium - 160 calories (kcal).

- Mars bar 33.8 g - 152 calories (kcal).

- Crisps, 1 pack - 130 calories (kcal).

- Whole Milk, 300 ml - 195 calories (kcal).

Now, the next stage is to consider what you can easily take out. Just one of them. Nothing more than that. It is all you need to get significant results. Once you have decided, you need to decide if you are removing it completely or replace it. If you remove it completely then you are dropping your daily calories by the amount of that item. Let us look at the banana as an example - 105 calories per day. That is 735 per week, that's 2940 per 4-week month. That will be a massive 38,220 in a year. Do you think for one second you will not lose weight from that? It is that easy to gain weight, and it is that easy to lose weight. One banana a day. You can stop at this chapter, try that, and you should be fine with your weight for the rest of your life. Hopefully, you will find the other chapters useful, too. Let us look at the option of change with the previous examples. You may have to do a little research for your alternatives.

- Banana, medium - 105 calories (kcal)

- Alternative - Satsuma - 50 calories (kcal)

- Latte, medium - 160 calories (kcal)

- Alternative - White coffee, large - 30 calories (kcal)

- Mars bar 33.8 g - 152 calories (kcal)

- Alternative - KitKat, 2 bars - 105 calories (kcal)

- Crisps, 1 pack - 130 Kcal

- Alternative - Popcorn, 17g bag - 76 calories (kcal)

- Whole Milk, 300 ml - 195 calories (kcal)

- Orange juice, 200 ml - 86 calories (kcal.

Now just doing one of these minor changes could save you a minimum of 50 calories per day, 350 calories per week and 18,200 per year. Again, a significant amount which will bring you fantastic results. Simple, easy, and once the change is in place. You just have to keep that as your habit. You can tweak this to suit you and you can go a bit higher if you want. But it should be more than enough. Needless to say, it will take time for the results to show. Most weight comes on gradually. This is a way of reversing that and taking it off gradually. I would estimate that this would deliver between half a stone to a stone per year. Which is pretty good considering no gym and no diet? Just a minor change.

Step 2 - Alcohol

Any changes you can make for the positive in this area will benefit you so much. It will greatly depend on your current consumption and with the changes we can make moving forward. The ideal amount is zero and nothing more. If you are having more than that, then I want you to ask yourself, why? People drink for the social aspect, some because they like it. Others out of habit. What I want you to do is to find out your reason. Once you find it and have a better understanding of why, then we can move onto doing something about it. Alcohol has no real benefit for the consumer. It may relax you, sure. But there have to be other options out there for that. It will give you a comprehensive list of health problems if you keep drinking throughout your life. It is basically produced by companies to take your hard-earned money from you. That is, it, that is the sole aim. They do not care about your health. That, my friend, is on you. So, 1 pint of larger is about 500 calories, give or take. To put that in perceptive, that is the equivalent of an average sized meal. If you have 5 pints or ten in a night, then multiply the calories. A scary number indeed. So, you can quite simply put in place a reduction here. You could also swap out what you are consuming for an alternative with fewer calories.

I want to consider the options of why you drink, social, habit, like it or maybe even partner drinks. There may be other options that I have not listed here. What can you do about these points? Social - you can reduce how much you go out for a drink. Now if you are going out once every 6 months, then you have no issue here. If it is more than that, then reduce it down. If you do not drink at home, then great, go to another chapter. Habit - think about it. Do you want to change it? Then what are you going to do about it? Like it, what alternatives can you find out there? Partner drinks, then you need their support if you do not have it. Then you have another issue. You might need a different book for that. Once you have identified the reason and considered your options for dealing with it. You then need to plan the dates that you want to implement it for, including start date and then a review date. 4 weeks is a good start. Take it easy and see how you go. Clear your body as much as you can from the toxins and reap the benefits.

Step 3 - Desserts

A lot of people love this course of a meal. If you are having a dessert at home, then you have not had a big enough main meal. It is just pure greed to eat more, not hunger. Which should be your first reason for eating. There should not be a second reason. Maybe to enjoy the food, sure. You can enjoy your main meal on its own. If you are out for dinner and you are working through courses. The simple option is to have a starter and the main. Dessert can be left and maybe replaced with coffee or tea. The whole concept of eating dessert is a massive barrier to success with weight loss. Your aim on this step is to eliminate or replace completely. Now you can have a dessert and you can enjoy it. But you must know how many calories it has; it must be strictly limited occasions. Now I am talking once a month and if you do that, then you need to record it on a calendar. Also, it will be instead of say having lunch, you will go straight to dessert. It will not follow a meal and it will not be an evening meal. These points are critical to your success. The other options you are presented with are having a dessert which is not high in calories. I do not think for one second you need me to tell you what a healthy dessert looks like. If you are a person that loves dessert so much and you cannot implement any of this right now. Then I would suggest moving on to a different step and maybe coming back to this one last. In fact, you may not even need this step. If the others help you enough, then you might be able to afford to skip it. You can make that decision later on and balance the enjoyment of dessert against what you want with your goal.

Step 4 - Breakfast

The first meal of the day. The classic saying it is the most important meal of the day. That was an advertising campaign created by one of the world's most famous cereal makers back in the 1940s. The problem is the message stuck and people still believe it. I get it, if you are in the army, a road worker or doing any physically demanding job, then breakfast is a great idea. But if you are not and you are just sat at a desk or driving a taxi etc, then you have more freedom.

You can take one of two approaches with breakfast. You can either have it or not have it. In order to get good results, if you are not having it. Then your first meal of the day will be Lunch, this should then be between 12:30 - 13:30. Try not to deviate from that too much. Another way to look at it is that you eat lunch about 5-6 hours after you wake up. After this you can eat all the way up until 9 pm, then repeat. In the morning, you can drink as much water as you need and up to 2 hot drinks. Hopefully, all of that is fairly straightforward and not too much of a change. If it is and you want to keep breakfast, then let us look at that option.

The option of having breakfast, you probably fall in to one of a few categories. These being cereal, toast, cooked or a healthier breakfast like Continental. This could be fruit, yogurt, or some modern-day Instagram image, like a fruit bowl. If you want results, then clear all of them off the table. Only one of them is staying and that is good old-fashioned toast. it goes back quite far in history before we even knew what obesity is, so if that is the case then you are safe. If you keep to two slices, do not overload the spread. You can put what you want on it within reason. I am not talking Nutella every day. The spread cannot be the same every day. You will have to change it at least once a week. You could have butter, jam, peanut butter, Marmite, or any other option you can come up with. Hold off from topping it with anything fancy, like fruits. That will increase the calories by too much. Pick a reasonable sized slice of bread for your toast, white or brown. That bit does not matter. Try to find one with a slice around 100 calories (kcal), that is fairly normal. But some go a lot higher. If you can find bread without lots of additives too, then even better. Try to avoid ingredients like tri-triglycerides. You will find these in almost every loaf on the supermarket shelf. There are only one or two that you will find that do not have them. This might be slightly challenging indeed. Spelt and rye are normally safe and maybe a few other options. A bread maker might be a good idea. Although that might present you with large slices and endless nice warm, irresistible bread. So be careful with that option.

Step - 5 Lunch

This section should not vary too much based on other elements of the book. It does not make much difference if you are working, at colleague or at home, etc. The same theory will work for each, and you should be able to put in place it, regardless. You can go with two options here once again. The first option is making your own lunch, the second is buying it. Fairly straight forward. One strict rule, you cannot have hot food for lunch. After that, you have real freedom to do as you please. There is an exception to the rule, if your evening meal is not going to be a cooked meal or a hot meal. Then you can switch them over and have a hot lunch. One hot meal per day.

When you are buying your lunch or even making it for the day. There is a limit to how many items of food you can have, which is four items. So, for example, a sandwich is one item, a packet of crisps is one item and so on. You can add on a drink such as a bottle of water, squash, tea, or a white coffee. No juice, soda, alcohol, milk, or fancy coffee for lunch. Unless it is a once a week treat. This can be a Monday pick up or an end of week reward. If you are making your lunch, then make sure you have it planned out for the week and that you have everything at home for easy preparation. Keep it simple, keep it varied and make sure it is food you enjoy or at least like.

Step - 6 Dinner

This area is a minefield, with so many options and variations. To keep it as simple as possible and easy for you to put in place. It will follow a similar process to the other steps. Where you will only have one or two simple rules or changes to put in place. This is mainly coming down to limiting or removing a few types of food. It does not involve removing whole food groups like carbohydrates. That alone is a silly move and a highly recommend you never do that. Right so when I say limiting, that means you can only have that food option once every two weeks. The foods you need to limit or remove are any meals that have cheese in them or remove the cheese. The other one, any meal that has chips or remove the chips. So, if you like cheesy chips, it's thin air for now. Just kidding. After this, you have fairly free rein to do as you wish. It goes without saying that you should not go mad about what you do.

Now takeaways are another ball game all together and have a different rule. There will be more on them under that step. But for now, the rule is no more than one a month for dinner and you can break the no chips or cheese rule, but that must fall within your once every two weeks. It is not an addition to that. To support this step, if you are having a lot of takeaways, then I would advise to go onto the takeaway step. You may even want to look at the step on lunch, but it is not really needed.

Step 7 - Supper

Rule 1 Stop eating 2 hours before bed. So, if you go down at 11 pm, then you stop eating by 9 pm. This includes any high calories drinks such as alcohol, milk and so on. A cup of tea or herbal tea or water etc is fine. Other than that, you have pretty much free rein over what you eat and drink during all other times. A big consideration here is, why are you eating it? What is your mood? How are you feeling? Try not to overload and eat unnecessarily. Now, by all means, eat, do not go without, and do not feel like you can't have it. Just take some control over it and do it for the need of eating. Rather than for the sake of it or out of boredom.

Two supportive measures you can put in place to counter the overloading of evening food are low calories snacks. Such as grapes, popcorn etc. See the Snacking step for more information. The other step is to make use of your hands instead of wasting time on TV, smartphones, or any other screens. Creative hobbies such as drawing, colouring, Lego building or even puzzles like Sudoku or crosswords. Maybe even games such as chess this could be done on a smartphone as well. So not always a bad thing.

If you want to take an extra measure here, then you could opt to avoid high-calorie foods. This could include chocolate, crisps in large quantities, sweets, cakes, and biscuits.

Step 8 - Snacks

You can use this section alongside the previous steps, or you can use it as a standalone. A rule with snacks is to either go with eating what you like and limiting it. The other option is to change them up and eat lower calorie snacks and eat as much as you like. As they say, you cannot have your cake and eat it. It is one or the other for this section.

If you are going with limiting the snacks, then it is four a day. It does not matter when you have them. So, the later in the day, the better. A snack cannot be a cooked meal, a bowl of cereal but it can be toast, up to two slices. It can pretty much be anything else. Use your sense with this. If it feels wrong, then it probably is wrong. A large bag of sweets or two donuts is going a bit far. Everyday snacks that most people would consume. Try to keep each snack around the 100 calories mark if possible.

If you are going with healthier snacks, then you can eat as much as you like. If you are not sure if it is healthy, then the answer is no. If it consists of fruit and veg, then you are fine. If it is labelled as healthy, then be cautious. Anything in a packet is normally dangerous towards your progress. At the end of the day, you do not really need a book to tell you what foods are good, and which are bad. You just need guidance around the

consumption and managing it. Keeping a balance and helping
you to make the right choices by being provided with some
information about it.

Step 9 – Water

The straight to the point guidelines state about 2 litres of water a day. I am pretty certain few people follow this rule. Although regular gym goers may hit that from carrying a water bottle around and refiling it a few times. This guideline is by no means bad or wrong. In fact, if you can hit that amount, then great. When they say 2 litres of water. I believe they mean in any form. Not just straight water. If you are having two cups of coffee or tea in a day, that is almost half a pint (quarter of a litre). Which should be included in your daily count. We will cover tea and coffee in more detail on that step and that section may also touch on water. For now, we will stick to the point of this step. Let us say just plain water or water with squash added. The amount you should aim to consume is 1 litre per day (2 pints). One at lunch and one at dinner. All other drinks will add to your amount. So, consume other drinks if you wish or increase on this amount to bring your water intake up to 1.5 litres.

Making sure you get the right amount of water will insure you have sufficient minerals in your diet. It will also ensure that you are operating efficiently, thinking right, and keeping you in a good mood. This is one of the most important steps in the book. To consume this amount as a minimum. It will not only contribute to your results. But it will also help you feel better and to feel good.

Step 10 - Coffee, tea, and hot drinks

Here we go, my favourite topic. Who does not like a nice hot drink and all the different varieties? Some really important rules in this section if you want to succeed. Now, I do not care if you do not like it. If you want to get into shape, then you must have at least one cup of coffee a day. I am not talking latte, with milk or anything like that, I am talking straight up black or espresso. Real coffee, with real caffeine. Try on the other side to limit your coffee intake. No more than 2 per day to get yourself to an optimum level. Make sure the last one is by 4 pm.

A cup of tea you can go mad with if you want, but do try to keep it below 4 per day. Also, no adding anything to your daily cuppa like a snack or endless biscuits. I think it also goes without saying the sugar and sweater is a no go. You want results or not? Make a choice. Herbal teas are quite simply unlimited. Hot chocolate is treat territory. Which means once every two weeks worst-case scenario. The other rule if it is not already clear. No cappuccino's, no lattes, no mocha, or any other fancy hot drink with a fancy name. Basically, a high calorie bowl of milk in a mug with an expensive price tag. This is your fast track to weight gain or failure at weight loss.

Step 11 – Protein

Do you need it well, yes? But not as much as you may think. Do people survive without it? Yes, they do, so that quite clearly defines that you do not need as much as you may think. The marketers will have you believing that you need it every 3 hours. They would, they make a lot of money from that. Does consuming high protein food really help with muscle growth. Not as much as you would think. Protein does help with the repair of muscle tissue and growth; it also has other roles. Can you get enough from a non-meat diet? Absolutely. If you have meat in one of your meals in the day, then you are getting enough protein. If you have a large bowl of cereal with milk, then same again, you are getting enough.

The actual balance of nutrients that make up your diet as a percentage would for protein be 15%. That is it. You can increase it up to 20% but not really needed. That is a small amount. The rest is made up of Carbs and fats, which we will cover on those steps. That figure alone should help you to understand how much you really need. Protein does help you to feel full, so if you are the type to always feel hungry, then it could be helpful for you in that instance. The calorie content of protein is also slightly less than fats but the same as Carbs at 4 calories per gram.

Make no mistake, protein is of benefit. But there is no need to go overboard and over consume. A basic tip is to eat 1-2 sources of protein per day as a minimum. This can be non-meat if you are vegetarian or vegan. You will also find the is plenty of options in that area too. You will not go short. If you want to be in great shape, then stop with the supplements. These are produced in labs, are full of chemicals and have more ingredients than processed food. The more ingredients in any food than the worse it is for you. Hence Apple, nuts, Carrot, etc. All one ingredient. The more ingredients, the more processed, the more calories. The bigger and unhealthier you will become. The one and only tip for this chapter cut the supplements. Eat real fresh food and it least 1-2 sources of protein per day.

Step 12 - Fats

Following on from the last chapter. Fats make up 25-35% of the diet. That is almost double the amount of protein. These numbers are not set in stone, and you could reduce or increase as per your individual requirements. Fats carry the higher rate of calories per gram at 9. So, the same number of grams of protein or carbs will be providing you with fewer calories. This should give you the simple and obvious information that too much fat will increase your size because of the higher calorie content. What can you do about it? Most items of food have a label that displays if it is high in fat. You are aware of it, so look at the label when buying food and then make a choice when you see that it is red and high.

If you really want to succeed in your quest. Then you will have to take massive and consistent action to eliminate high fat, high-calorie foods. Despite the fact it should make up a large portion of your diet. Most people are consuming high amounts of fat and calories. So, make it a high priority to take control of these two areas. Put a number on the high-fat foods you consume and then try to reduce them by one a day. That is a simple and easy start. No more is needed than that and you can increase if you need to make more progress later on. You should see results with just the one change over the next four weeks. But if not, one more drop and then you will four weeks later.

Step 13 – Carbs

Carbohydrates (Carbs) are an essential nutrient for your diet.
Forget what any other diet book states. Carbs are heavily present
in vegetables, which are one of the most natural foods on the
planet. You will also find it in other foods such as bread and
pasta. In which case, you should not consume as much. The
recommended amount is about 50-55% of your diet for
carbohydrates. Some guideline uses a plate for reference. If you
had a plate of food, then only half of it would have pasta, bread,
grains etc. Which for some this would reduce the portion of this
nutrient.

The primary function of the nutrient is to give you energy. If you
limit it, as other books advise, then you will end up feeling tired,
lacking energy, and suffering from headaches. Does that sound
healthy to you?

When it comes to your meals, use that as your guidance, half the
plate maximum. If you are having more than that, then you
should get progress from this step. On top of that, any snacks
which are carb based should be only 50% of your daily snacks.
This includes cereal, beer, crisps, juice, chips, etc. So, reduce
accordingly. Test it and review after 4 weeks. If no progress,
then reduce by half again. No more than that. After that, move
onto another step as an addition to this section.

Step 14 – Vitamins

Vitamins are absolutely essential in your diet to help your body function. Vitamins play an important part in your body. The benefits include improved digestions, an efficient immune system, strengthen of the bones and improved circulation to name a few. The list goes on and on. Most vitamins can be obtained from your diet. Good sources include meat, nuts, seeds, fruit, and vegetables.

In order for you to get good results, and for you to succeed with your goals. You will need your body to be functioning the best in can be. To do this, you need all the vitamins in your diet at or slightly above the recommended guidance. You can do this through maintaining a balanced diet. It may be helpful to use a calorie counting app, as most of them display vitamins per food item. This will then enable you to see when you have hit your daily amount for each vitamin. It will also enable you to tweak your diet to increase or decrease each vitamin where needed. The easiest and sure-fire route to get all the vitamins you need. Without going through all of that. Is to take a daily multi-vitamin tablet. You do not need an expensive tub. Just ones that contain all the vitamins and have near to the recommended daily amount. That is all you need from this chapter. That is the key point, tip/step.

Step 15 - Supplements

Supplements are just that, they supplement your diet for any area that you may not have enough from food. For example, as per the previous step - vitamins. So, do you need supplements? The answer is specific to you. There is no generic yes or no. If you do not have enough of a nutrient or vitamin, then it may be worth taking a supplement if you cannot get it from food. If you do not know if you are short on a nutrient, for example, protein. Then it is pretty pointless to take a supplement. As you may already be consuming too much. In which case, find out how much you are consuming of each nutrient and vitamin by recording what you are eating and drinking. You can use an app if needed to make it easier. Then you will have an idea if you need a supplement. First, maybe try to find a food high in that nutrient or vitamin and go with the option first if you can. If not, then use supplements to support your diet. This should by no means be a long-term option. Most supplements are processed and not the best option for your diet.

The key tip here is to use supplement to support your goal but to do it with intelligence. Do not overdo it and make sure you know what you are taking and why you are taking it. Be smart about using alternatives. If there is a fat burner that you think will help, check out the ingredients. If the main ingredient is something like caffeine, then what is the alternative? Coffee perhaps?

Step 16 - Dairy products

Dairy products are largely milk-based products. Including yogurt, butter, and cheese. All of which have a good amount of protein but also have a high amount of fat. Now for guidance on fat head over to that step if you have not already. I think without any guidance you already have a good understanding of fat consumption. If you do not, then it is something you should consider reducing if you are consuming high amounts.

The steps you should aim to implement in this chapter are limiting dairy products during main meals. Reduce this as much as you possibly can to get results. This would include milk consumption, so for example cereals. The other main element for this section is to ensure you only have dairy in about 1 in 3 of your snacks. The alternative here is to have dairy in each snack, but only a 3rd of each snack can be dairy.

If you need to increase your protein consumption, then dairy should not be your preferred choice. Due to the fat contents. Aim to make that increase from other food groups. This could be from meat, fish, nuts, grains, and pulses.

Step 17 - Sweets

When we say sweets here, we are talking about the bags of sweets or packets of sweets. We are not talking about all sweet foods such as cakes. That will be on another step. This is for everyone's favourite that we grew up on.

Now I am hoping in general that you do not consume sweets on a regular basis. If you are, then a review is needed immediately. When I say regular, I mean weekly. If you are having them this often, then reduce it to every two weeks. If you are in two weeks, then down to once a month. If you are having more than once a week, aim to get down to once first of all. The key point here is a reduction, and not a small one at that.

The number of calories per packet or even per sweet is really quite high. For such a small item of food that will provide you with little nourishment or even meet your hunger needs. In which case, the key reason people eat sweets is because they like them. It is a treat, and everyone should have a treat now and again. But let us just keep it at that, every now and again. You do not need the high sugar content in your diet, and you do not need the high calorie content. The final end target is no more than once a month.

Step 18 - Chocolate

Every item of food can have some good benefits and there is always some backing for cocoa. The key information missed, though, is that chocolate does not contain a great amount of cocoa. You will also find the benefits are heavy outweighed by the high levels of butter, sugar, and fat in chocolate bars. Now you can get standard bars of chocolate with higher levels of cocoa. These can be slightly better for you considering the higher the content, the less room for other ingredients.

One point I want to get across to you that chocolate can really push against your goals. A single bar that breaks into squares, those small little squares. 3 small squares can contain around 100 - 150 calories. This may vary depending on the type and size. If you look at the single serving bars of the self, they will be about 100 - 250 calories.

I would not expect anyone to really eliminate it from their diet. Considering in the shop there is such a range of choice. This gives you a great opportunity to find an alternative bar from any usual one you might have. In which case, you may be able to go from a 200-calorie bar to a 100-calorie bar. If you have 4 in a week, then that is 400 calories a week and 1600 calories a month. Have a look at your consumption, make a small change and see some great results come from it.

Step 19 - Cakes

If you have come to this step, then it is probably because you like a cake. Now you are not alone with that, a lot of people do. The bad news is they are one of the worst foods you can consume if you want to get results. The reason is and you will know this if you have ever baked a cake. They contain a large amount of butter and sugar. Which equals high fat and high calories. For which you know what happens from there once you consume it.

This step is to establish how much of a problem you have in the first instance. Write it down what you are eating in this area. It could be as easy as looking at your shopping receipt. You may have to make a big change in this section if you have them a lot.

One thing you can do is to find an alternative, a sweet food with fewer calories, sugar, and fat. If you are a big fan of cakes and just cannot eliminate them. Then you need to learn everything about them. How many calories, how much sugar and how much fat they contain. Plus, anything else that might help you. Find out what the best option is, and which one will help you to get the results that you want. You want the lowest calories, sugar, and fat for your cake. One that you will enjoy eating but will not cause you any harm with the results you crave.

Step 20 - Biscuits

This step follows on quite right from the previous step of cakes. Now the reason for that is they both have very similar ingredients. They are also very similar with how they affect your body and health. A packet of biscuits can contain an unreal number of calories. If there were two foods, you need to remove from your diet. It would be without a shadow of a doubt, cakes and biscuits. The main other culprit for people being overweight is alcohol. Go to that step for guidance in that section.

The guidance for this step is similar to the cake section. If you have a lot of biscuits and really cannot cut them out. Then you need to learn everything you can about them to help you get the results you need. One biscuit alone can contain around 50-100 calories. Again, it depends on the size and type. Think about that for one second. Let us just go with the lower number of 50 calories. How many biscuits would you consume in one go? Let us just say 5 for augment's sake, that is 250 calories. I am sure some people could consume 10 with ease and probably do. That is 500 calories. You get the picture, that is the equivalent of a large main meal. What would you rather have from a portion's perspective?

Your preferred choice of biscuit can easily be substituted for an alternative with less calories. You can also make a reduction in this area with ease if you are consuming 10 in one hit. Just dropping two per time will save you about 100 calories. That should be enough to get good results.

Step 21 - Takeaway food

The first point you need to do here is to look at how often you are having takeaway food. Some people have it 2-3 times a week, maybe more. Some have it once a week, every other week. Some once a month and some none at all. If you are only having a takeaway once or twice a month, then move on. You have no problem here.

What I want you to do if you are having it every week or more is to think about why? Do you have it because you like it or because you do not know how to cook? There must be a reason, find it. It may even just be a habit. That is the first thing you need to do. Work out why? Once you know the answer, it will help you to work on the prevention of it carrying on.

The step is for you to answer the question, can I reduce it by one or replace it with something else. If you can reduce it by one, then see what the results are like after one to two months. After that, reduce again if needed for greater results.

If you can replace it, then can you cook a healthier alternative. If not, then why not? Look at recipes, find an easy one and then give it a go. I bet it tastes nicer than your local takeaway food. If not, try another recipe until you find one that does and one that you can cook well.

Step 22 - Eating out

Now this section may not be too much of a concern depending on where you eat out. If you are eating in fast-food restaurants, then go back a step to takeaway food. As it is basically the same principles for fast-food restaurants.

As for eating out anywhere else, restaurants, for example. It comes down to the places, types of food and amount of food. When you go to a restaurant, some of them will have a menu that displays calories. If you find this, then you are onto a winner, as you can use it as a guide to make sure you are not overeating. Try to keep your meal below 500 calories, including your drink. This may mean no alcohol. You can vary this depending on the occasion. If it is a regular occasion, then take some control. If it is a one-off birthday or similar, then fine. This means your birthday, not everybody else's birthday.

If the calories are not displayed, then you are on your own. You will need to make a decision and you will want to make the right one. In order to help you do this, the rule is you cannot order anything that you could easily make at home. The main ones to avoid include pizza, burger, chips, and fried breakfast. As you can easily put any of these dishes together at home. Which means if they are easy to make, then they are highly likely to be made. So, avoid eating these kinds of meals when out. Go for the dishes you cannot do at home and cannot do well.

Step 23 - Peer pressure

Why would someone pressure you into making a decision?
Normally a decision that is the same as the one they have made.
Because they want approval, it makes them feel significant, and
it provides them with a connection. As someone is like them and
doing what they do. When someone is putting pressure on you,
then they are doing it for themselves. They are not doing it for
your sake. You need to check yourself if you are making a
decision based on someone else.

What you eat and consume is your choice and your choice only.
People may judge you for it, bully you for it and everything else.
No matter what your age or background. This happens, and I
have been in this situation on more than one occasion. Never
again. Now I have full control and so should you. One of the
best ways to tackle this is to not even share your decision with
people. If you have made your choice, you do not have to
communicate it to anyone. If they do not ask, then do not tell.

If they do ask, then do not give a straight answer. Make it
difficult for them to get the information out of you. Turn the
question back on them and ask them what they are having or

doing. This may even come back to you. The longer it takes you to decide or even share then the less chance they will try to influence your decision.

If you are presented in a difficult situation like this time and time again with a certain person. You may even find a person is always trying to put pressure on you or influence you to doing what they want. Then you should aim to spend less time with this person. If the person is someone, you are close to all, like spending time with. Then you should communicate to them how you feel about it and that you want it to stop. If they cannot accept this, then you may have to cut someone out of your life. Now that is a big decision, but what comes first, you or them?

Step 24 - Juice

When we say juice, we are talking about fruit juice. In other words, juice that is made from pressed fruit. Such as orange juice and apple juice. We are not talking about fruit squash which is diluted with water. The reason I have put that explanation in is that it can have different names in other countries.

The fruit juice you find in the shops may come from one of two locations. The chilled section, being the fridge and off the shelf, non-chilled. It does not make any difference which you buy. You will also find concentrate and not concentrated, also it does not make any difference. One thing that does make a difference is that almost every juice on the shelf except orange and apple. Contain a large number of additives and additional ingredients. To add flavouring, to save on the cost of the fruit they are trying to create the flavour for. So, the only juice you should really touch is apple and orange. Maybe even pineapple in some cases. Check the carton before buying. If it has more than one or two ingredients, then you do not want that in your body. The main point from this step, though, is that juice contains a high number of calories. To reduce this, you could swap it out with a squash that you add water to. If you do not wish to do that, then take a look at the calories you are consuming from each cup. Then make a minor reduction over the week. You could do this by having a smaller glass or taking out one day a week of having it.

Step 25 – Milk

The unusual thing about milk is it comes from animals, and we drink it. They produce it for their babies and we have it as adults. The main reason we do this is because it is high in nutrients, proteins, and fats. It is cheap, easy and can be used in a variety of ways.

It would be reasonably easy to eliminate milk from your diet. If you can manage taking out the foods that are produced from milk. Make no mistake, there is no real need to remove any milk-based foods or drinks from your diet. They are reasonably high in calories and fat, so any reduction may help you.

The other thing with milk and milk-based products. People can have reactions and the can be numerous other health implications from consuming these foods. If you feel sluggish or do not feel great, then this could be the cause.

You may have milk in your coffee with cereal or consume a regular amount of yogurt, butter, or other dairy based products. Which would be the easiest way for you to get results. Take out the option that you find easiest to remove. If you can go without milk in your hot drink, then great. If you can swap out cereal for toast even better. It is your choice. Make a small change and run it for one to two months, then review it. See what the results are like. Take measurements, weight, or anything else you want to check when you come to that review.

Step 26 Movement

Movement is included in this book, along with some other sections on exercise. This is due to how much they can support your results. How much do you currently move? Movement is the single most important thing for the body. After the essential operations that happen automatically and the consumption of food and drink. It is like the food and drink side, whereas we have control over it to some degree.

You should be moving regularly, but do not overdo it. Aim to walk one to two times a day. At least 15-30 minutes over each walk. If you currently do that amount, then increase it by 15-30 minutes.

Every aspect that you can increase your movement the better. If it is walking to work, hoovering the house, or cutting the grass more, then doing it. It will help your base level of cardio fitness; it will help improve breathing capacity and it will burn extra calories. How you do this is up to you. It is another small change in your life, but it can make a big difference. Especially from a health point of view.

Step 27 Exercise

If you already exercise, then great. But are you doing effective progressive exercise? It is not a case of just showing up and doing something. Although that is a good start. To get results, you need to make it progress over time. This can be a gradual increase in the time you train, the intensity, or even the amount of times you train.

Whatever exercise you choose is up to you. Make sure you it is something you enjoy. Something that you will look forward to doing. Even if you do not enjoy exercise, full stop. There will be some form out there that will work for you. You may just need to find the reason to enjoy it. Be it the benefits, the social aspect, or the adrenaline release. If you do not, then it will go quickly. You will stop or give up in no time. Something enjoyable with help you to build consistency and we all know consistency builds results.

Whatever choice you come to for the form of exercise you want to do. Make sure that you are doing it at least 2 days a week, as a minimum. Aim to hit 3-4 if you can. If you go as much as 5 days a week, then expect great results. Train for up to 6 weeks at a time. Once you get to 6 weeks, then it is time for a week off. A break or rest is always needed. It will help your body to recover in a lot of ways and it will also help you to progress and come back strong.

Step 28 - Stretching

Another element that will contribute to the overall aspect of what you are looking to achieve. Any kind of goal in relation to diet, fitness, and health. All lead back to one ultimate goal and that is good health. To be free from any health problems and to be as healthy as you can be. So, in order to do that, you need to look after yourself in every way you can or even know how to do so. With that in mind, one of the best options is to look after your muscles and joints. These are basics that assist in the movement of your body. In order to maintain efficient movement, you need to maintain flexible muscles and joints. The most effective way to do this is through regular stretching. A range of stretches covering a full body routine is best. Ideally, you want to be doing this every day, that's right, 7 days per week. You could have a day off and just do 6 or whatever you can manage. The time frame does not have to be a lot. You could get away with 10 minutes a day, maybe first thing in the morning or last thing at night. You could even do both. If you can provide or make a routine that works for you, then great. There are some really good yoga platforms out there, including live classes. If it helps, then start off with 1-2 sessions a week and then build it up. You will find over time that being more flexible will enable you to move more freely. It will reduce muscle tension and inflammation. It may even eliminate aches and pains. Finally, you may find it helps you to improve and have a better posture. All of this will help you towards a healthier lifestyle by far.

Step 29 – Weightlifting

This step outlines what you can do with weightlifting to assist you on your journey to success. Weightlifting can give the most return for the least effort. What I mean by this is that any training you do has a lasting effect. The lifting of weights breaks down muscle tissue and as it repairs over the next few days. Your body will continue to burn calories. In which case you are get more from it than just the day of training you put in. You will also increase muscle density, which helps to burn more calories. It would be unlikely that you would build muscle size. As that can be very difficult to do. People train for years and do not get the size they desire.

You will find it has a greater benefit in weight loss than it does in building muscle. The guidelines are to get in 3-4 sessions per week for a good amount of progress. More session than that will bring you results quicker. You could get by with 2-3 sessions per week. Less than that, then you are not really ready to start.

When doing this kind of training, it is best to complete a workout that covers all the major muscle groups. It can be in one day or split over a few days if you get to a more advanced workout. This can bring with its other benefits, including a lower resting heart rate, increased lung capacity and increased bone density.

This will not be the easiest step in the book to implement, as in involves a real lifestyle change. It also involves a big-time commitment. But it will really help you to succeed and can also provide you with a hobby.

Step 30 - Cardio

This step can assist you with any weight management due to the high number of calories you can burn per session. This will vary depending on the type of cardio you are doing. It will also be affected by how much you weigh and the amount of time you are training.

The various options include running, cycling, cross-training, rowing, punch bag and a range of sports to name a few. You can test out different options to see what you enjoy. That should be the main factor of your choice. You should also consider any effects on your health and your ability to actually take part. If it is high impact like running outside and you are carrying knee injuries, then you may be better off with cycling. This can also help then strengthen that area. Another area you could look at is which is the most effective area for results. So, for example, a punch bag can provide a higher calorie burn per hour than, say, cycling or rowing.

In general, an hour of cardio can burn up to a good 500 calories, depending on the different variants. That alone is a good amount. Now you may find it easier to eat less calories than to burn them. That choice is up to you. The guidelines recommend doing at least 2-3 days a week at a moderate intensity.

Even if you do one 30-minute session a week, that can be about 200 calories. Which will help you to get results. As that is 800 calories a month. Which can make a big difference over time if you keep it consistent. It is not a short-term fix; it will be a lifestyle change. Something that you enjoy and can keep doing ongoing.

Step 31 - Exercise classes

This step leads on from the others around exercise and is to really outline how it can help with your goals. The aim is to also to give you a basic idea of the options out there and the benefits to you. We will also cover as per the last few steps how much, how often and suitability.

Different options out there include circuit training, aerobics, indoor cycling, Pilates, and yoga. Most classes run for a time of about an hour, in which case will give you a calorie burn of around 500 calories. Depending on the type of class, how much you weigh, etc. Different classes come with different benefits. Such as yoga working on flexibility. Pilates on core strength. Aerobics on cardio fitness and circuits on muscular endurance.

The amount you do falls in line with the guidance on weight training, cardio and stretching, depending on which class you are doing. Ideally, aim for at least 2-3 days per week for good results. More if you are doing yoga or stretching based work. Any increase will provide you with some benefit in the long run. Be it an improvement in heart efficiency, lung efficiency, or flexibility. Which class you choose again comes down to what you think you will enjoy, but also be aware of the impact on the body.

Step 32 - Calories

The almighty calorie is the main contributor to any weight gain or loss. It is the key element. Take control of this and you will have control, full stop. There are certainly other aspects that come into play, but nothing as important as calories.

Calories are a unit of measurement for the energy that we use and consume. Consume more than you need, and you will gain weight. If you do not consume enough, you will lose weight.

To work out how many calories you need. You take your weight in kilograms and multiply it by 25. For example, if you weighted 90 kg, you would do 90 x 25 = 2250 calories (kcal). This gives you 2250 calories per day as a base amount. If you were active, then you would add a percentage on top of that to maintain weight. sedentary then adds 25%, moderately active then adds 50%. Highly active, then add 100%. Moderate would be 2-3 days per week exercise. High would be 5-6 days per week exercise and maybe an active job. So, for example, if you were moderately active, it would be - 2250 + 50% = 3375 calories (kcal). If you wanted to lose weight, you reduce it by up to 500 calories. 3375-500= 2875 calories. If after 2-4 week you have not dropped any weight, then reduce by a further 100 calories. Then review every 2-4 weeks. Take in mind your weight might change, in which case review the calculation. Never go below that base minimum of 1200 calories. You can log your daily consumption of calories to stay in line with the figures. This can be done either through using a calorie app or good old pen and paper. This is a highly effective method of managing your weight. To lose or gain weight as you please and to have it under control.

If you were to use any step from this book. This would certainly not be the easiest, but it does work. No one ever said it would be easy. But if you want great results, then this step is worth the attention.

Step 33 - Sports Drinks

Sports drinks, energy drinks or anything else similar. They all contain sugar or sweetener. Which means if it is sugar, then they are fairly high in calories. Some energy drinks can contain around 100-200 calories on average. This is in the same region as a soda drink, for example, a bottle of cola. The reason they give you energy is that energy is normally sugar. The ones with sweetener have alternatives such as caffeine. Any of these drinks, even if they are labelled for sports, are not really any good for your goals. If you are running a marathon or some high endurance event, then it may be beneficial. As you may need the energy to help you through the event. If you are trying to reach a goal, then they will only have a negative effect on your training. Having a sports drink in the gym, you may as well have a bottle of cola.

If you consume any of these drinks, then find out the reason. If it is because you believe what they advertise to you. Then fine, you now know different. If it is for the taste, then find a replacement. Something that you know will not work against you. If you can work them out gradually or take them out completely, then great. The best alternative is straight up water. If for whatever reason you cannot manage that, then find something low calorie that works. The less sweeteners and additives they have, the better. The fewer the ingredients, the better. At least have one glass of water per day, whatever you do.

Step 34 - Veggie + Vegan diets

This subject made it into the book based on two reasons. One, it has been a popular topic over the past few years. Two, it is an area that I have lived and experienced. That is really the only knowledge I will be bringing to this step. Sometimes that is the best knowledge, something that someone has lived. Rather than just learned. From that experience, I found that meat free diets can be the best and healthiest diets out there. As long as you cook your own food and avoid any processed foods. The basis here is that the majority of the foods are heavily based around vegetables and grains. The main issue with meat-based foods is they have a lot of fat in them. You will find any reduction in the area of fats will benefit you.

If you have a meat-free diet or similar and manage it well. Then you will see the benefits, including the large range of vitamins and nutrients. Which will help you to feel great and be a lot healthier.

If this is a step that you already live, then great. Your step is to make sure you are cooking your meals from scratch as much as you can. If you do not have a diet like this already and want to give it a go, then your step is to try it for a week. If that works, then go 2-4 weeks and see how you get on. Once you have done it for a while, you will start to see the results.

Step 35 – Fruit

Fruits, as you probably know, contain a good amount of nutrients and vitamins. There is not much in the way of negatives to come with the consumption of fruits. If you want to be in good shape, then there are a few I would limit or even avoid. These are avocado and dried fruits. I would also limit bananas to no more than one per day. That is your real key point to put in place for this step.

The other point which is added benefit. To ensure you have at least two pieces of fruit per day. This will help you ensure you are getting a good range of vitamins in your diet. Which fruit you have is up to you. Just follow the guidance above on what to limit. Try to vary what you have in order to get a good range of vitamins in your diet.

After that, you are all good. Do not mix this section up with fruit juices. See that step for guidance. The information provided to have 5 per day is inclusive of vegetables. Note to remember this is also a minimum amount that is recommended, so by all means have more. When you have them, during the day is up to you. It would be advised to consume them up until about 4 pm. After that you should not need so much sugar. Albeit with natural sugar. The time may vary depending on your circumstances. For example, you may work nights. So, vary to suit your needs. If it helps, then log your daily eating habit for a week and then review it, at the end, to see how much you are eating and how often.

Step 36 - Vegetables

The guidelines for vegetables come under the 5 per day as a minimum. This varies by country. Aim to hit that amount however you do it. There is no upper limit. In other words, consume as much as you want. Similar applies from the fruit section. Try to eat a good variation to provide your body with a range of vitamins and nutrients.

This could be the easiest or hardest section for you. If you are already consuming enough, then you do not really need to make any changes. If you are not consuming enough, then it can be really hard to increase it. So, what can you do? The first step is to find veg that you like, and you know you will be able to consume easily. Even if you are just having one type, then fine. It is a good start.

Try different methods of preparation, so you could cook them in different ways if you do not like one way. You could have steamed, shallow fried or even oven baked as a good range of different methods that can provide tastier options. The traditional boiled option often leaves them tasting tasteless and with not the best texture. Even if you end up eating raw carrots, fine if it works for you.

Step 37 - Nuts and seeds

Nuts and seeds are definitely a good source of nutrients. There is also a really varied range of options out there. They also come high in protein, which has its benefits. But they also come high in fat, and they also come high in calories.

They could be put into a category alongside avocado, dried fruits, and juices. Generally, really good for you. But they all contain so many calories that they will have a real negative effect on your achieving results. There is no harm in consuming them, they can all bring a great range of benefits. But if you do, then keep it controlled and limited.

I would recommend not having more than a handful of nuts and seeds any more than twice per week. Now this is all depending on you and your circumstances. If your calories are low and you need to increase them, then this can be an effective way of doing it. It is also a good way to increase your protein intake or fat intake if needed. One big caution, as per all packaging, is to avoid at all costs if you have any allergies. Consult a qualified dietitian before making any drastic diet changes. If you are not sure, then do not take a risk. There is a big difference between dietitian, nutritionist, and nutritional adviser. Only the dietitian can provide you with qualified guidance.

Step 38 - Eggs

This one is one of the old age debates. Are they good for you or not? We'll let us have a look at it. They say cholesterol is bad for you and eggs are high in cholesterol. The is that point, and it is best to keep it down. In which case, the aim here is no more than twice per week. Up to 3 eggs per time.

They are also high in fat, protein, and calories. Which for 2 out of the 3 backs up the point of keeping the consumption down. Now they are high in protein and that can be of some benefit to you, but it is outweighed by the other points.

So, the key step here is to keep your consumption under twice per week. This will help you to keep down the calories, cholesterol, and fat. If you need extra protein in your diet, then there are other ways of getting it.

The eggs that you consume, should be cooked in the healthiest way you can. If you are cooking with any kind of oils, then you will be adding calories and fat. The better options are poached and boiled. Which will avoid that problem.

Step 39 - Planning and shopping

This could be one of your key steps to getting results and making sure you do not fail. Great success with a lot of things comes down to planning. In which case for this step, plan out your shopping list. Write it down, on a notepad or on your phone. If it is not on the list, then you do not buy it in the shop. If you are making all your meals from scratch, then you will need to list all the ingredients that you need first. Then get them on your list. Make a list, stick to it and then you will only have in the house what you need.

When it comes to the shop, the aim is to go straight to the sections based on the list you have created. Do not even look at other sections of the store. Cross off each item on the list and do not pick up anything else. The aim of the store is to sell you as much as they can from every section. They want you to buy the high processed foods because they make a lot of money from it.

Once you have some recipes that you find easy to make and are quick. Then all you need to do is list out what you need and keep going with it. Take one step at a time, do not change too much too soon.

If you live with other people, then you will need their input. It will have to be agreed to save any falling out. Once agreed, then proceed. Take in mind other people may not have the same objectives as you. In which case, have an open discussion at the right time about the support you need. If you cannot get the support, then you may have to go it alone. Make it clear that it may happen. Then follow it through.

Step 40 - Food preparation

Food preparation is a large key to success. If you have this in place, then you will always be prepared. In order to prepare right, it helps to get a good understanding of how often you eat, when you eat and what foods are best for you. Once you know how often, then you know how much food you need to prepare. Once you know when, then you can prepare for those times.

The foods that will be best are foods that you like, help you to feel full and are easy for you to prepare and transport if needed. This may take a bit of time for you to find and to work out. But it will be worth it. As you will always have the right food with you at the right time.

In order to prepare your food, first start with making a list. For your list, make sure it covers all your meals, snacks, and drinks. Once your list is complete, then plan out what containers you may need for any work or travel. At this point, before you prepare any food, you will need to consider the life span of the food. Plus, any storage instructions, such as chilled, etc. Then work out how many days you can realistically prepare the food in advanced. Prepare the food at a time that suits you and on a suitable day. Make sure you store it correctly and mark it if needed with dates or any other information such as day of use. You have all this in place, then you have everything you need to progress. Good food, healthy food at your disposal when you need it.

Step 41 Food Labels information

The label on the back of a packet tells you all you need to know about that item of food or drink. It will have the ingredients listed highest to lowest in regard to content. So, for example, if sugar is the first word on the list, then there is more sugar in it than anything else. You will also find the information for each nutrient, including weight in grams and calories (Kcal). This will give you an indication of how much fat, carbohydrates and protein are in the product and which is the majority in the product.

All information is normally presented per 100 g of the product. Take in mind the item of food or drink may be less that that or more in volume or weight. Sometimes they display the information for the size of the product, but they do not have to do that. The 100 g is so you can have a standard comparison against all other products. Some drinks will display it for the size of the bottle or can. These things may vary by country. This information can also be useful for you to get an idea of how many calories you are consuming, which helps you to measure a total over the day. You can go to the calorie chapter for further guidance.

It will also help you to make sure you are not consuming too much sugar, salt, fat or any other nutrient or ingredient. You may also find information around suitability for allergies and dietary requirements, such as a vegan diet.

It is exactly what it states information, and it is there to make sure you are informed. Use it and have it to help you guide yourself in the right direction.

Step 42 - Meat

Meat within your daily recommended guidance should only make up about 1 meal per day. It should be no more than half the meal. Ideally less if you can. The once per day is really the maximum too. If you can have it less than that, then great. Your first choice should be white meat, no red meat. Red meat should be less than once per week. Due to the high levels of fats and the other risks that it poses. You will find a lot more of the red meats are processed too.

Meat is one of the highest forms of protein, but not necessarily the best. Also, your need for protein is only about 15-20% of your diet. In which case, there is no great need to be eating meat on a regular occasion. The only benefit is to the people selling it to you. If you like meat and want to consume it on a regular basis, then that is up to you.

The guidance here is to make sure you are not going over once per day with consumption. Then no more than once per week for red meat. Each time you consume it, then no more than half your meal. Meat really should be considered as a treat. Too much of it has the potential to cause health problems.

Step - 43 Fish

Fish comes under a similar category to red meat. It should not be consumed too often. The guidance is about twice per week as a maximum. Fish has a lot of benefits, including high levels of protein and Omega-3. Now the amount will vary depending on the fish and the size of the portion. They also contain fats but not as high as most meats.

Generally speaking, fish is a good option to have in your diet, providing you have no allergies. If you think you do not like it, then have you tried all the different options and the different cooking methods. Oven baked will be one of the best options from a health perspective. Tried to avoid deep fried, but a treat once in a while never did any harm. I am talking no more than once a month here. Then shallow fried is a good go between option. It can be quicker than over baking, but needs more attention. When it comes to baking, you can just wrap it in tinfoil, surround it with prepped veg and bake it for the required time.

If you do not like fish and do not want it in your diet, then you will do just fine without it. Move onto another step. If you are eating more than the guidance, then look at replacing with an alternative.

Step 44 – Fasting

Fasting is not always necessary, but can help you to get past a plateau. It is always helpful for a quick win or some fast results. It is worth noting that fasting should only be short term. I would not do it for any longer than a period of 4-6 weeks. I also would not follow any guidance ongoing days without food. The fast should only be up to about 16 hours. For this, you could quite simply stop eating around 21:00 at night and then eat again the next day around 13:00. This can reap many benefits, including easing bloating, decreased body fat and improved health. The time you do this does not really matter.

It is flexible. You just really need to hit the duration. The remaining time frame, you can eat as much as you want and whatever you want. Although I would advise that you treat your body with respect and provide it with nutritious food. To back that up even more, if you want good to great results, then you should be doing everything you can. So, do not use the flexibility as a reason to overindulge. What it does for you really is ease the pressure and any worry about what you eat and how much you eat. So, it is a kind of takes away a lot of the process and makes life easier for you. If you go with the approach of, I can eat anything and everything, then you are setting yourself up to fail. The key point is to go a period without food to let your body digest and process the food and drink you have consumed and to clear out any toxins. Give your body a chance to recover and to stabilise. 16 hours, including your sleep time over a 24-hour period. This leaves you with 8 hours of eating time. In theory, you are just skipping breakfast. Which is not the most important meal of the day. Do some research and find out where that saying comes from. You will then realise that you have been sold to by an advertising campaign for years. Do not believe everything you hear and read. You do not need to have breakfast. You just need enough energy and nutrients for each day.

Step 45 – Food swaps

Whatever you are eating, you can normally find an alternative. The alternative you are looking for is one that has less or more calories. Depending on if you wish to gain or lose weight. Most people have certain items of food that they consume on a regular basis. This may be a certain breakfast or snack. Such as a certain cereal for breakfast. The snack could be anything from a piece of fruit to a bar of chocolate or a packet of crisps. So, what can you swap them for, well almost anything? You are looking on the packet at the kcal (calories). Look it up if it does not have it on the item, such as a banana. If you have a Mars bar every day or 3-4 days per week at around 229 calories, then you are looking to swap it for something with 50-100 calories less. This could be a KitKat at 106 calories. Saving you over 100 calories a day. In which case, a lot over the next 6-12 months. It may be a banana at 110 calories and swapping it for an apple at 60 calories. These numbers can vary depending on the size of the fruit. But you get the point. It is a case of changing one or two things in your diet to help you get big results over time. Now if you go back to the old item of food, then you lose. It is not a short-term fix. If you want to get results quicker, then you can start to look at your whole diet. If you go to one burger chain over another. Check the comparison of calories in their burgers. You may even find switching in the same restaurant from one type of burger to another. Such as comparing a quarter pounder to a big mac. If you go through and make changes with your whole diet, then the pounds should start to drop off quickly. If you are looking to gain weight and switch up the calories, then you should gain weight quickly. This can all be affected by your current weight, age, and metabolism. Once you have made the changes, then you are up and running. All you have to do is to keep them going as a habit and not to change back. This can be done by making a list before you go shopping and then sticking to it. By getting anyone, you live with on side. If you do the shopping, then you are in charge. Do not be weak and let people bully you into getting out of shape. If they want something, then they can have it. Then you have to be strong by not copying them. As that is what we do, let other people copy you and win the game.

Step 46 – Food diaries

A simple method of recording, seeing, and analysing what you eat. You may think you know what you are currently eating. But you do not really know how many calories you are eating over the day. The amount of food you eat is not really relevant. What matters is the number of calories. These can be logged in the diary. Record every item of food and every drink that you consume and then note how many calories each item contains. As you go along, make a running total and a final total for the end of the day. You will need to find out what your limit is by taking your weight in kg and multiplying it by 25. Example 25 x 100 kg = 2500 calories (kcal). Add a further percentage depending on how active you are, 25% for non-active, 50% for moderately active (training 3 days a week) and 100% for highly active (train 5-6 days a week and active job). So, for example 2500 + 25% = 3125 calories (kcal) per day. Now if you wish to lose weight, then take off anywhere up to 500 calories, so 3125 – 500 = 2625 calories. Every 2 weeks recalculate and then lower if needed. As your weight will change. If you do not drop any weight, then lower it by a further 100 calories after 3-4 weeks. Then repeat. Never drop below 1200 calories. If you are on that low an amount due to being a low bodyweight, then you may not need to lose any weight. Workout your BMI online with an online calculator and make sure it is not below 19. If you are, then it may be worth considering increasing your weight, which can be done with weight training and an increase in calories. Which should actually make you in better shape but at a higher weight. Because really, the weight on the scales doesn't count for or mean anything. It is just for guidance and if you are in the healthy range of BMI 19-25 and the healthy range of body-fat, then you have nothing to worry about. Good health should be your goal. Not getting obsessed about body weight. Once you are in the healthy range, enjoy your life, keep a good balance to your diet and if you wish, then you can exercise to tone up. Once you have got to a goal weight or BMI range etc, you can stop the diary and just come back to it if needed. The only reason this may happen is if you change your diet again after getting the results.

Step 47 The feeling from food – before and after

We go through a range of feelings throughout the day. These can be happiness, anger, stress, joy, delight, and a range of other feelings. Sometimes these can be affected by how you eat, what you eat, or even the amount that you eat. Sometimes you may even eat in order to change your mood, to make yourself feel better. It is the classic tub of ice cream trick when feeling low. Some people may even binge eat as a comfort thing due to previous incidents in their life. It may even be because you do not have anyone with you. It may even be your parents gave you food whenever you were upset as a child. These things could go way back, beyond what you can even remember. The key to this step is to raise awareness of what you do and why you do it. Only you will know the answer to that. In order to do it, log a food diary and write down how you feel before and after each item of food or drink that you consume. After a week, look through it for patterns and reasons why you may be having that coffee first thing in the morning, that glass of wine last thing at night. You get the idea. Once you find out, the reasons for some of your consumption is beyond needing nutrients. Then you can plan alternative replacements or even eliminate them if possible. One thing you can do here is to find another way of dealing with the problem. If you are having a coffee to wake you up in the morning. Can this be rectified by making sure you are getting the right amount of sleep or by starting your day with a cold shower or some tai chi? You get the idea. Make healthier habits, find out what it is you are doing, and then fix it. You may even find that you can use foods to make your life a little bit better. So, if you are feeling down a lot. Can you use some nice foods that you like which are not unhealthy to improve your mood? Be careful doing this as it can snowball and cause problems, such as eating disorders. So only do this with good, healthy food. Doing it with clear decision making and do it with a plan in place. Make sure it is only to your benefit and only to make your life better. Consider the pros and cons and how it may affect you after. So still log it, log how you feel and if it helps. Then review it after 4 weeks, look back at it and analyse any trends.

Step 48 – Eating on holiday

This step is very straightforward. If you are going on holiday for no more than 2-3 weeks, then you do not need to worry about making many changes. The reason here is that any damage you do once a year on a 2-3-week holiday will quickly be reversed when you return back to normal. The problem is, if you are going on multiple holidays per year. Anything that is giving you consistent increase in the consumption of unhealthy foods or high calories foods and drink. The other area to be cautious with is if you go away for 2-3 weeks and you make a regular habit with a change of consumption. This could lead to you taking it home with you and continuing with the wrong choice on a regular basis through habit. So, the key step here is to not bring home any changes to your diet that are unhealthy or high calorie. Quite an easy step if you do not come across any big changes or you do not make any. It may not be the type of foods. You may find that you are eating out more or drinking more. The other issue with this step is if you exercise regularly, then it may break that routine. It may cause you to stop training upon your return. As I would advise to stop training on holiday, it is a break, and it should be a chance for your body to recover. You could reduce your training or do light training in order to prevent the routine from being broken. If you are aiming for great success and do not want to go off track, then you should keep as close to your regular diet as possible. Alongside this, if you maintain the implementation of 3 -4 steps from this book over a 4-week period, then you will continue to see results rather than regress. The key points here are to do what will work and what will get you results. If you are following the steps of the book over set 4-week periods and you want to have a break from it and change your routine, then that is your choice. But you live with your choices. So be warned. Your aim is to get results, so do what will get you results. If you do take a break, then get back on the 4-week cycle of implementing the steps.

Step 49 - Benefits of healthy eating

There is a great range of benefits from healthy eating. This comes from having a good nutrient, vitamins, and minerals. So, in order to reap the benefits, you need to make sure you are getting all of these in your diet. Quite simply, consume at least 2-3 pints of water per day, that is a minimum, add flavour if you need to and it is not high calorie. One multi-vitamin tablet and split your meals with a good amount of carbs, fats, and protein. At a percentage ratio of 50% carbs, 30% fat and 20% protein. So, half of your diet is carbs, just under one third is fat and then one fifth is protein, just in case you need a conversion. Aim to consume good carbs and good fats. Not starchy carbs and saturated fats. You may need to do a little bit of extra research for this step if you are unsure.

These elements have all been covered in previous steps. For this step, you have to implement all 3 of them and you can't do them alongside the other steps that incorporate them. By doing this, you are supporting your body to being in an optimum state and getting the health benefits that come with it. Including an improved metabolism, decreased body fat percentage and reduced risk of ill health. It will also help you towards your goals and you may even experience other benefits such as improved mood, clearer mind, and less stress on the body.

If you find it hard to implement all of these at once, then do it gradually over a period of time that suits you. For example, you could do one per week. Starting off with increasing your water intake. Set 3 reminders on your phone for throughout the day, reminding you to have a pint of water. The following week, start your daily multi-vitamin and then, after that, start planning out the balance of your nutrients.

Step 50 - Keeping a balance

Keeping a balance to your diet is vital for good health. Having a balance of all the vitamins, minerals, and nutrients. The is government guidance on a balanced diet, including the Eatwell plate and the previous model being the food pyramid. Both reasonably indicate how you should balance your diet. The ideal situation is that half your diet is fruit and vegetables. Grains, pulses, nuts, and seeds can come into this area. The other half being fat and protein. These are less vital than the carbohydrate-based foods. This all makes up the first part of this step. Know what balance you need. Consider the changes you may have to put in place to meet this part and then move on to the second part of this step.

The next part is to keep a balance to the foods that you consume. Now, despite years of knowledge and experience built up from working with clients, education and testing out different things with my own diet. This tip comes from a relative of mine. You can eat anything in moderation. It is when you eat it frequently and/or in a large quantity that you will start to affect your health. A way of doing this could be to track what you consume. An easier way is to limit each item of food you consume by 1-2 per day. For example, 1 packet of crisps, 1 apple, 1 chocolate bar. If it is a large size item, then pay attention to the portion size and only consume 1 portion. This applies to all foods and drink, so no more than 1 beer, 1 burger and so on. This alone should give you a reduction in your calorie consumption. It will prevent over consumption and help you to keep a balance to what you are eating. If you can and want to take it to the next level, then limit it over a 2-day period or even more, as high as you can go. So, for example, you may only consume 1 alcoholic drink per week or any other type of food or drink, except for water or healthy foods.

Step 51 - Mind and thinking right

A lot of what we do, including eating and drinking, comes from one place. The mind, it can also come from what we see, hear, smell, feel and taste. Quite simply, the senses, which lead back to the mind. I would estimate about 80-90% of what you are currently eating, and drinking comes down to habit/routine. As you are on autopilot. Your mind has so many tasks to deal with throughout the day that it is easier to not decide or think about it and to just do it. The same as last week. The remainder 10-20% as an estimate is influence, by advertising, what you see, what you smell, what your friends or family are eating and drinking. Either that or you just fancy a change.

Here we need to get you thinking about what you are doing to make new habits. You can either write a daily list of what you are consuming, or you can reflect on what you know needs to be removed from your diet and what you know needs to be added in. If you do the list, it then leads onto that same point of analysing it. The next part is to make a shopping list. You can only buy what is on the list, no changes allowed in store. The exception being something essential. If you see something you want that is not on the list, then it will have to go on the list next week. No impulse buying, think about it for a week and if you have forgotten about it, then it is not important.

The next part is to think outside of your home consumption and to reflect on what you are eating and drinking when you go out. Be it at work or visiting friends and family, etc. How much do people influence you and how much can you take control of that? Reflect on the changes again that you know you want to make. What will be best for your health, goals and moving forward. Write it down, what you are going to do and when, then use it as a plan for each week. Make small changes first and then review it every 4 weeks. Including checking results.

Step 52 - Body and taking care of yourself

The true element of health and wellbeing is to live free from health issues. To do this, you will need to look after yourself and your body.

Starting with your mind, give it a rest from the daily grind of work, play, social media, tv or anything else. Give yourself a break from everything for at least 10 minutes per day, even better if you can do 10 minutes every 2-4 hours. Just relax and stop, appreciate life. Let your mind switch off from everything and just enjoy your surroundings. Also look after your mind by using it, read for 10 mins a day minimum, play a game which involves thinking such as sudoku or a puzzle of some sort. It can be anything which gets you thinking. Again, 10 minutes is fine. Do something for you, which helps you relax. Limit any negativity around you by being careful who you spend your time with. Do things that you enjoy but are also good for you. Take time twice per day to think about the great things in your life and the great things about you. It can be the same each day if needed. If you cannot find any, then think about what would be great and then write it down. Then write down how you can make it happen or what you can do to make it happen. Once you get there, then you have that to think about daily. This will help you to feel gratitude and will help you to live a happier day, each day that you do it.

Next is the body, utilise daily stretching for 10 minutes, movement including walking, tai chi, or yoga. Clean daily everything, look after it as it is the only one you have, your body that is. Treat yourself with the utmost respect and you will be so much better in all areas, including mentally. Avoid the consumption of any toxins, chemicals, alcohol, or anything else that may have a negative effect on you in any way. Limit high calorie, high fat, and high carb foods. Provide your body with clean nutrient-dense foods, including a large number of vegetables, fruit, grains, seeds, and low fat/lean meats. Drink water 3 times per day minimum, with each glass being round 500 ml.

Step 53 - Downtime – preventing burn out

Downtime, a break from whatever. Be it work, life or whatever consumes a lot of your time. This can also apply to exercise and healthy eating. So, if you are training 5/6 days per week, then every 4-6 weeks give yourself a break, or whenever you feel you need it. If you work 60 hours weeks, then give yourself a nice two-week holiday at least once a year. You get the idea. Now when it comes to eating right and living right, looking after yourself. If it is easy and comes naturally and it is not an issue for you, then keep going. Especially if you feel great and look great. If you have not made it that far yet and everything you are doing is a struggle, then give yourself a break every now and then. It must be a scheduled break to prevent you from going back to your old routine. In which case plan a break every 2 months from any areas that you are struggling with. Review how things are going, consider any changes you would like to make and plan out the next two months of how you are going to live, eat and drink. During the break, I would plan it for no more than 5-7 days. During this time, you can do whatever you want, whatever works for you. All I would advise is do not lose respect for you and your body. Treat it with respect and look after it. Do not go over the top with consumption and quantity. You are only looking to break from the routine, to freely eat and drink as you please for the short period of time, while you reflect on your success, what you have achieved so far and what you wish to achieve moving forward. Consider going through Step 56 – reviewing progress at this time if you feel it will help you. Generally, you want to reflect on what you want, when you want it by, and how you are going to do it. Basically, a plan of action.

Step 54 - Goal setting

Goal setting should be simple, effective, and setting the course of action towards the end result. In the instance of this book, we are goal setting for your dietary habits. Changes that you want to make and that will benefit you in the long term for your health, wellbeing, and shape. We could follow the standard SMART acronym. Specific, measurable, achievable, relevant and time bound. Instead, we are going to go with my adaptation. What do you want, when do you want it and what are you going to do to get it? Quite simply if you know that you are eating too much chocolate, biscuits or drinking too much alcohol, then you already know the change that you need to make. If you do not, then start with a diary of what you are consuming and then look back at what you are having a lot of over the week. You could even just look at your shopping list. So, you know the change. How soon do you wish to achieve this change and for how long are you going to maintain it? That second bit is important. You can set in place a change and probably do it easily, but that might just be for a week. In which case commit to a time frame such as 4-8 weeks and then treat yourself to that item of food or drink at the end, then review the goal and set another time frame. The goal has to progress, you can't review it as in do it for another 2 weeks. You would have to do the same time frame or more and then add in something else, another item of food or drink that you wish to limit. So, we have the plan and the time

frame. What are we going to do to make sure this happens, to get
it, to win the game? In the case of making a change to your diet
is to look at where it starts, is it the supermarket, is it the
shopping list, is it friends wanting you to go to a certain
takeaway restaurant? Whatever it is, look at how you can change
it. Write it down. If all you have to do is write a shopping list
and stick to it, then that could mean that the item of food or
drink isn't even in your house. If you have to, then put an
alternative in place. But you get the idea, have a plan, then do it
straight away. Do not stop to think about it.

Step 55 - Body stats and measurements

Whatever you do and whatever you want to achieve. If you do
not have a start date, a target date and the measurements and
stats to compare, then you are working on guess work. You will
have limited hope of getting there. So, crack out the scales,
measuring tape or whatever it is you want to measure and
review. Write it down, log the date, line it up with your goals
and then review it every 4-6 weeks. Make sure you use it to log
small goals/steps towards your goal. Every measurement you
take, do it over 3 days, 3 times and log an average. Log the time
of day that you do it, so the comparison is equal. Measurements
you could take include bodyweight, body fat percentage, BMI,
and waist to hip measurements, to name a few. Use a range if
you can as one on its own may not give you a fair reflection of
the results. If you do not know how to do the measurement or
what equipment you need, then do a bit of research online before
making your choice. Choose the methods most relevant to your
goal, so if you want to reduce your waist, then take a
measurement at that point. If you want to decrease or increase
your body weight, then stand on the scales. If you have a high
level of body fat and want to reduce it, then you can use a set of
callipers and take measurements. Make sure you are taking the
measurements in the correct areas, and you use the same points
each time you retake them. The measurements you take are the
measurement of your success and will give you feedback on

how you are progressing. If you review them every 4 weeks and you do not get any changes, then that is fine. That feedback tells you that you need to make a change to your approach. If you keep going the same way, you will keep getting the same result. So, the next step for you to do is to read another 2-4 steps and implement them for the next 4 weeks. This should give you a level of success. In which case, keep it going until it levels out and stops progressing. Once it does, then add another 2-4 steps. Keep going with this approach until you reach your goal. If you reach your goal, then you need to make a new goal, even if it is to maintain where you are. This is relatively easy, as you should just keep doing what you are doing at this point.

Step 56 - Reviewing progress

We have touched on this step a bit throughout the book, but it needs its own chapter. If for anything really to enforce the importance of it. In order to move forward, you need a plan and, for the plan to be successful; you need to follow it. If you were to take a journey, you would need a map or GPS, in which case you would put the location down. To get there, you would follow it. How many times do you not do this and if you do, then do you ever end up going the wrong way and taking longer to get where you are going? Once you get there, you may review the location, as you may want to go home at some point. The same applies to your success with your body shape. You need to get down where you want to go, what route you will take and once you get there, where are you going next. Hopefully not returning to where you came from. An example, you want to lose 1 stone in weight (6.3 kilograms) about 14 pounds (lbs). The guidance is 1-2 pounds per week. In which case 4 pounds in a month, 8 pounds in 2 months, 16 pounds in 4 months. There you have a plan. After 1 month, you may be on target, great. If not, then you need to increase the number of steps you are following as per the guidance, 2-4 steps. The next 4 weeks will then give you progress. It may vary depending on the steps you pick and how well you implement them and any other changes you may make. The second you stop setting and reviewing goals and having the plan in place will be the moment you fail. You can choose to succeed or fail by either giving up or by keeping ongoing and reviewing and planning. Every 3 months, take a break, give yourself some time off. It may be the summer and you may have a 2-week holiday; it may be Christmas. Whatever it is, plan it in so that you can have 1 - 2 weeks off every 3 months. This can be varied but make sure it is in a diary, dates recorded and written down, as this will increase your chances of success by about 70-90%.

Step 57 - Personal trainers

During your journey of obtaining a diet that works for you. You may decide to support it with exercise, nutritional guidance, or support from others. A good way to hit or 3 of those points is to get a personal trainer. Now, this may not be essential, but it could be a good way to get extra support or to give you a kick start on your journey. Finding the right trainer is the best place to start. You will want to check they are qualified first; you can do this by asking to see their qualifications or you can check on the register in your country. This will show you they are qualified and is normally an online portal which lists their name, location and qualifications achieved. Once that part is covered, check the pricing of their service is right for you and your budget. Then proceed onto a consultation. You will know straight away if this person is the one for you, you will have a rapport and will get the feeling that they care and want to help you. If you do not get this, then book another consultation with another trainer. During the consultation, they should be checking you are fit to train, what you want out of it and planning out how you will get there. Hopefully, they will check with you what training you enjoy and dislike, what you have done and what has worked for you previously. If you are not getting this, then you may want to try someone else. Once you get to training, you should find the training hard, but not too hard that you cannot do it. They should adapt it to your needs, and it should be progressing over time. They should be focused on you and making sure that each exercise you do is safe and effective with plenty of feedback on performance and form. The goal should be established and worked towards with the plan, adapted as and when needed based on how you perform and the results you get. You can use a trainer for a phase 4-6 weeks or you can use them for longer. Maybe even until you achieve your goal. Maybe even beyond that, as you may establish a new goal if you achieve the original one or your focus changes.

Step 58 - Exercising at home

Exercising at home can also help you on your journey. If you can do it between 3-6 days per week, then you will increase your chances of success. This can be something as simple as going for a 30-minute walk. Now, if you are already doing that, then you will need to increase what you are doing. For example, the amount of days or the duration of the walk. The aim is to make progress and, in order to progress; you need to increase what you are doing. If you want to train in the house, you may need some basic equipment although you do not really need anything. A gym/yoga mat can be beneficial. One of the easiest and simplest forms of exercise is callisthenics, for example, bodyweight exercises. All you need to do is a full-body workout. For example, squats, press-ups, abdominal crunches, dorsal raise, Russian twist, and dips. This will cover a large area of the body, although you are limited with back exercises when it comes to bodyweight. Unless you have access to a chin-up bar. You can do 1 set or as many as you need depending on your fitness level. Each set you should aim to do 12-15 repetitions of each exercise. If you do more than 1 set, then rest 30-60 seconds between each set. You can switch out the exercises for other ones by doing a search online for bodyweight exercise. Just make sure you are switching to the same area of the body. If you take out a core exercise, then replace it with another core exercise. If you need to see how the exercises are performed, you should be able to find a video online, although watch more than one for each to make sure you are finding one with the correct form. When you do each exercise, if it does not feel right, then stop. You should only feel it in the muscle that the exercise targets and any muscles that assist. If you need guidance on this, then seek the guidance of a trainer. Any training should be done for a period of 4-6 weeks, followed by a week of recovery.

Step 59 - Cereals

Cereals have their own step due to the popularity of the food. They generally take up more space in a supermarket than the meat section and almost as much as the fruit and veg section. They have managed to produce a type of food that a large amount of the population consumes on a daily basis. They have also managed to convince us that breakfast is the most important meal of the day. People believe it and they do not even know where that statement comes from. It was an advertising campaign in the 70s by one of the largest cereal producers. What they did not tell you is that skipping breakfast brings a lot of health benefits. They also did not tell you that you can survive for days, even weeks, without food, depending on how much you weigh. Not to mention that in the western world you have food readily available at every street corner.

So, for this step, eliminate cereal from your diet, replace with an alternative such as toast or just stop eating it full stop. Remember, they feed cereals to cows to fatten them up. It really is not good for you. Not to mention they must pump the cereal full of vitamins to give you some nutrients from it. In taking this out of your diet, you will also be reducing your milk consumption. Which will help to reduce your calorie intake. It will reduce the intake of hormones from the milk. It will reduce inflation in your body and will help you to improve your body shape, reduce body fat and fat consumption.

If you like cereal and want to consume it, then it should only be consumed as a treat about once per week. If you can make it a healthy option such as muesli or porridge, then great, but keep in mind these are high in calories. In which case, they should also be limited.

Step 60 - Frozen food

Frozen food covers a wide area, most of it is fine. The same applies with all food, limit processed foods. Eat the foods with the least ingredients. Frozen fruit and veg is not much different from fresh. It might even have more nutrients in some cases. Meat if it is not processed and of good quality is fine. The flip side of this is that most supermarkets will use cheap cuts and low quality in the frozen section. If you are buying fresh food and freezing it, then you know what level of quality you are buying based on where you buy it and the price. It goes without saying that anything from the ice cream or dessert section is not going to help you on your quest to getting and staying in shape. So, cut it out, grow up and eat some real food. Rant over.

The key point here is you can buy veg and meat from the frozen section and it will not do you any harm towards your goal. As long as it isn't covered in batter or breadcrumbs. Even more so, if you buy good decent meat from the butchers and you need to freeze some, then even better. You can rest assured that it is local, good quality and you can buy enough for a couple of weeks to keep you going. The ideal situation is that you eat your food fresh, but we have the luxury of saving us from going out every day and saving time with a fridge and a freezer. Modern day life is great, but do not get slack on it. Look after yourself and treat your body with respect.

Frozen food can be used here in a simple way of having a piece of meat with a range of vegetables with very limited cooking effort needed. For example, a chicken breast or salmon, oven baked and supported with oven baked fresh veg or some quick boiled frozen veg. A very easy, cheap low-calorie meal. 2-3 times a week with a different meat each time will work wonders. You can even add a sauce if you wish.

The other key point to this step is to stop with the chips, chicken nuggets and all the other processed frozen food. Replace it with foods that are high in nutrients, vitamins, and minerals. Not only will you get results from this, but you will also start to feel better and look better.

Step 61 – Time

Time can be a factor in a lot of people's diets. So much so that the popularity of microwave food, takeaway/fast food and ready-made food is through the roof. People seem to think they do not have the time, yet not many people work more than 40 hours a week and this has not changed. The only thing that has changed is the options. You have the option to go with the quickest option, which was not there before. At least not on the massive scale it is at now. Where you can have any fast food delivered to your front door. If you lack time, then you need to start managing your time. Logging every hour of your day and making sure the top priority is you, your health and what you consume. If all of that does not come first, then you will not operate efficiently, and you will end up out of shape and unable to perform at an optimum level.

Easy options to get your food habits in order are batch cooking, cook a meal one night that you can box up leftovers and freeze them, building up a range in the freezer, so all you have to do is reheat in the oven or in a pan.

Plan out quick easy meals to cook, such as stir-fry's or oven baked meals that do not need a lot of attention. You can even go the slow cooker route.

Prep and plan out meals for the week or at least for 3 days to ensure freshness. Every 3 days tends to work well.

Make sure you have boxed up healthy snacks on hand to prevent impulse eating. Plan these out and look into all the different options and variety to keep it interesting.

You may find you are on the road a lot, or you may need to take food with you to work a lot. The same above applies. Have a decent lunch box, one that you would like to have and use. Plan out the contents and the variations to keep it interesting. Have more than one if needed, if you eat more than once while out for the day. Then make sure you do the same for a drink that you will be consuming. Ideally, make sure you have enough water throughout the day, but that is another step all together.

Step 62 – Travel

Travel as per the last step can make a big difference to you getting results or not. The key reason being if you are not prepared and do not have what you need, when you need it, then you are subjecting yourself to chance. The chance or risk of what food there will be wherever you are going. In which case you will have to decide on the spot of what you are going to eat. The choices may be limited and then you know how this will end.

The key point to this step is preparation. It rings a similar tune to some of the other chapters. You know where you are travelling, how long you are going. This then gives you an idea of how much food you will need. You can even check out the area and establish what the options are for you when you get there. If you are going away for a few days, then you may want to check out the area. If you can, then take a few days' worth of food. Keep in mind, you want fresh food that will not go stale. This can be challenging as most healthy food will go stale and most junk food is full of preservative that will make it last. This will be something you may want to research and find foods that you like that are not high calorie, high fat with nutritional benefit. If you travel a lot, then you should spend a bit of time on this in order to give you the best chance of success. Snack boxes with a range of foods that you like can be great. Just ensure they are balanced. As in, not a load of processed foods.

If you are only out for the day and you have not taken any food and the only option is junk food, then make a decision. Do not be swayed by the easy route. Remember, you can go for days without food, even weeks. As long as you have plenty of water, then you are not going to die. Do you feel hungry or are you eating just because of the time of day? It is lunchtime. Man invented time, so why do we eat on schedule? Who benefits from that? The people selling food. Eat when you are hungry and only then. Even when you are hungry, you can go through it and see what is like on the other side. It goes away. It will come back again and go away again. Now do not get me wrong here. I am not saying to go weeks without food. All I am trying to get across is you do not need to eat on schedule, and you can easily go all day without having anything if need be. Now if you are in the army, working a physically demanding job or running a half marathon, for example. Then you may want to ensure you have eaten sufficiently. Also, if you have very low body weight or body fat, I would advise making sure you are eating the average recommended calorie intake for the day. I also would not advice this for children that are still growing. This book is mainly aimed at adults, for which case we are talking 21+ as the body is still growing and developing until that age and even beyond. The key thing is if you are overweight, you haven't had breakfast; you are out for the day and the only option is burger and chips, then you will be fine waiting until you get home, even if it is late.

Step 63 - Eating for reasons

We eat for a lot of reasons, including hunger, enjoyment; you see something that looks good or smells good. You may be in a social gathering with food readily available. You may be feeling down, or happy, and then certain food may follow. You may associate a certain food with an experience in your life. I can remember when I was younger eating a desert when we were out for the day. I then went back to this place about 30 years later with my daughter and they still did the same dessert. Needless to say, I had to re-live that experience with her and it was great; I loved the experience, but the dessert was nothing special. It was when I was 8 years old, but at 38 years old; it was average.

The point to this step is to get an understanding of why you eat what you eat and when. As if you know why, then you can take control and make changes if you feel it is necessary. As in, you may not want to eat something and you are just doing it for routine. But you may want to eat something if it is for the experience. Spend a week or two writing down what you eat and the time of day, then next to that log, how you feel or why you feel you are eating it. Then add to that do you need it or just want it? 9 times out of 10 you should be writing want it.

Once you have this guide in place, you will have the insight into what you are doing. You will even receive immediate feedback, as you may see that the reasons are not aligned with what you want and then you may change what you are doing on the spot. Otherwise, if you don't, then read back over it after the week or the 2-week period and then start to write down against each time that you have eaten what you would rather have eaten or what you can do instead of eating. Then use this as a drafted plan to guide you with your next food shop. Alter and perfect your diet to the point you are eating because you wish to be eating. The most dangerous to your goals is eating for habit or even taste. Make it work for you and make sure that the most of your eating times moving forward are for the need of food and nothing more. It does not always have to be that way and you will want to eat for the experience or enjoyment, but this should not be every day, maybe not even every week.

Step 64 - Implementing your plan

Whatever your plan turns out to be like, you will need to implement it. You will need to take action to get it off the ground and to get results. Your plan starts before even picking up this book. Which is a bit backwards, as you may need to read this before planning. You can read, learn, plan, and then implement.

It starts with the goal and what you want. You probably already know this to some degree. It is always worth spending a bit more time thinking about it and reviewing it, even if it is in your mind. You then need to write down the process you will follow to get to that goal. It can be short and even better if it is just bullet points. This makes it easier for you to read, understand, and to follow. The more you can have planned out, the better including the steps you will take to act. This should include planning everything into each day, which might be times that you eat, what you will eat, and where you will eat. Do you think having those things written down will make a difference? If you have a guide on where you are eating, a time and what you are going to put in your mouth, Sure it will. If you doubt it, then try it and prove me wrong. Keep this guide close to you like it is your mobile phone. Not on your phone, but on a piece of paper. Does losing weight or hitting your goal mean a case of life and death to you. Well, in could be, you just may not know it. In which case, keep the plan on you like it is a matter of life and death. Open it every time you are thinking about eating, then just read it. Fold it up, keep in the back of your phone case. Easy. Oh, and do what it says. It is your plan. No one is telling you what to do on that plan but you. Now that plan you may need a bit of guidance on, in which case you will need to review other steps in the book. Goal setting, planning, and shopping, and calories may help you. This step is all about putting it into action. Sometimes, beyond what we have covered, the easiest thing to do is to stop thinking about it and to just do it. Stop sitting, stop thinking and to just do and move and do and move. Be obsessed with it and be relentless. The results will be amazing.

Step 65 – Barriers

On everyone's journey, the will always be barriers. Barriers can be anything that will prevent your success or limit it. This could be not having enough time. It could be your family cooking a meal that does not align with your aim. It could be that you are working a 12-hour day and do not have adequate cooking facilities or a fridge. This list is endless, and everyone has different barriers that will get in their way. Like other steps in this book, find out what your barriers are. You do not need to write these down. Just go through a normal week and see what prevents you from taking the route that you want to take. Once you know what your barriers are, then you can do something about it. What I want you to do here is to take 10 minutes out of your day, even if you sit in your car in the car park. Somewhere away from everyone, the family, friends, your kids, etc. Then take this 10 mins and think about what you can do to get past these barriers. As if these barriers are the only thing preventing you from success, then 10 minutes may be all you need to work out what you need to win.

Some questions to get you thinking, rather than giving you all the answers. As with a lot of things in life, you will not find the answer from anyone else. The answer is within you. As no one knows you better than what you know yourself:

- How can I manage my time?
- Who can support me with my lifestyle changes?
- What can I do to prepare for success?
- How can I make it cost effective?
- How can I make my meals and snacks healthier?
- What changes can I make.
- How am I holding myself back?

You may find that there are more questions relevant to you, but this is just to get you thinking. You want your life to flow, and you want it to flow with ease. Which is why we make a lot of the decisions that we do. So, whatever you are planning to put in place, make it easy for yourself and make sure it will flow. The brain does not like to think too much as it has so many other tasks to do, so make it easy for your brain. It is also seeking pleasure, so try to manage that with small doses of pleasure from food rather than regular high amounts.

Step – 66 Results, winning the game

Results can and will come. The only reason you will fail is if you give up. So, whatever you do, keep going. As with life, you are not working towards a final point. You are not looking to get somewhere. As if you are when you get there. It will be over. In which case, then you may end up going backwards. Which is fine. It is just part of the journey. Do not beat yourself up about it. Everything in life is temporary, nothing is permanent. One great thing I have learnt in life is that it is not about the situation you are in, it is how you deal with it. If you are in a situation that you are not happy, then deal with it the right way and you will make it better. If you deal with it the wrong way, then you know where it is going to go.

The key point to this step is that if you hit your goal, no matter what it is, then what do you do next. This point has been echoed throughout the book. Whatever you do next needs to be something you want to do and something you will enjoy, as without those two elements, you will most likely fail. The planning and reviewing steps help with this, but the key is to find your next step and to have something in place to motivate you, to give you purpose and to help you to keep moving forward. Because if you do not then, not only may you stop doing what you are doing, you may also relapse back to how it was before. A way of preventing this is to review your steps that were successful and plan them out again. Keep yourself around the people that have been supportive and the people that have helped you. Some people will always encourage you to go off track. You do not need them doing that. Put a stop to it. Review any planning or diary management that you have had in place and making any changes that you may need. You can also go back to any new steps in the book if need be or any that you have not done yet.

Summary

If you manage to implement all 66 steps, despite any that may go against others as they may not all work in harmony with each other. You are sure to get great results. Everyone is different and everyone will need a different number of steps for success. This can depend on your weight, height, activity level, lifestyle, and a range of other factors. If you get to step 66, you may even need more to keep progressing. But I assure you, we have covered a wide range of areas and most people will see great changes if they get as far as 66 steps. Although you may only need 1 to 4 steps for great changes in your life and sometimes that is enough. Pick the ones that suit you, tailor them to you and your diet, ultimately there is no wrong or right. What works for you is the best way to go. Give it time a period of 4-8 weeks before reviewing and making changes. Remove what does not work and keep doing what is working. Because if you keep doing the same thing, you will keep getting the same results. Most importantly, enjoy it and live your life.

About the Author

After writing my first two books, which were non-fiction. Based around areas of knowledge and expertise. I gained throughout my working career and through further research. I decided to have a go at writing a novel, something I always dreamed of doing. Throughout the process, I discovered my love of writing fiction. This led to self-publishing my books and completing every process, from editing to cover design. I continue to this day as an independent author. Writing alongside working full-time, parenting and volunteering. Along with the other challenges of life.

My main focus is to give as much as I can and to help as many people as possible I can. Give people stories to pull them away from the normality of their day. But most important to enjoy every step. If any of my books or work have helped you or if you have enjoyed them, I would love to hear about it. As that it what makes it so enjoyable. Thank you.

For more information

Contact: BenjaminHarris@gmx.com

Thank you.